THE
SILICON
VALLEY
BONUS
SYSTEM

THE
SILICON
VALLEY
BONUS
SYSTEM

A BRAND NEW WAY
TO GET THINGS DONE

Incentivize Your Team Without Creating a
Runaway Monster Bonus System that
Will Eventually Wreck Your Practice

DR. CHRIS GRIFFIN

The Silicon Valley Bonus System
A Brand New Way to Get Things Done
Incentivize Your Team Without Creating a Runaway Monster Bonus System that
Will Eventually Wreck Your Practice

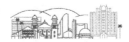

Images provided by Presenter Media.com

Printed in the United States of America

First Printing, 2018

ISBN 978-0-692-18048-8

Dr. Chris Griffin

415 East Walnut Street
Ripley, MS 38663
(662) 837-8141
www.SiliconValleySystem.com

CONTENTS

DON'T FORGET YOUR FREE BONUS TRAINING WEBINAR

Register for your bonus training that goes with this book by going to **www.SiliconValleyBonus.com** On this training, you will learn:

- How to **identify a Death Spiral Bonus** before it makes everyone miserable and kills your team unity

- How to apply the Silicon Valley System to your Practice in a way that could <u>double your practice and make your team love you for it!</u>

- You can **stop spending THOUSANDS each year with big marketing companies and slick consultants** who try to convince you that your results are better than they actually are.

- This is THE MISSING PIECE of the training for Implants, CEREC, Ortho, or any other highly advanced skills you have acquired. I <u>don't even think you should do those trainings until you learn this protocol.</u>

- This is THE answer for the age-old problem of doctor›s not having enough time to manage their team. **The Silicon Valley Secret will turn you into a Lunch Hour CEO** (and it won›t even take nearly the whole hour.)

- Once Your team starts seeing how this makes the practice better, THEY WILL LOVE YOU FOR IT!

  Go to **www.SiliconValleyBonus.com** and sign up today

PROLOGUE

It's 9:15 on a Tuesday night in May 2013. I'm standing in the rain with a handful of my friends and family members. We're watching the dental practice I built with my own two hands burn to the ground.

It's strange to watch an event that you know, in the moment, will alter all your hopes and dreams. It makes you think. It's the kind of soul-wrenching experience that removes the façade you have built for everyone to see. It forces you to look deep into your heart and mind for the next steps you will take when you're ready to move forward.

When the path you have been traveling is not only blocked but ripped up and destroyed, you feel despair, sure, but you also are finally freed to pursue and create something special. It's the ultimate do-over, and precious few are blessed with the chance to hit that reset button in the middle of their professional journey.

That night I turned my gaze inward and discovered that while my outward success was fleeting, the core upon which I had built my success still lived. I decided to take that core and work to perfect it. It was time to rebuild not only my practice but also my professional existence.

Sixteen months later, I unveiled the first edition of my dream practice for all to see. It is now—and forever will be—a work in progress, but it reflects my hopes and dreams in a way that is more true to my inner passions than ever before.

Let me share just a few of the ways my life is better thanks to my dream practice becoming a reality:

Peace of Mind – The Silicon Valley System ensures the myriad important procedures for making a practice profitable and successful are being completed. These critical tasks are not only getting done, they are being implemented in record time by team members who are eager to see the practice grow.

Less Stress – Before we implemented the Silicon Valley System and were driven by what I call a death spiral bonus system, there was always a lot of stress in the office. Tension quickly arose between team members when it looked like we were going to miss a bonus, and I think the patients could feel all the negative emotion, too. Nowadays, I almost feel like I need to stir things up from time to time just so I can relive those "good ole days." Just kidding!

Working Less Than Ever – We were already seeing patients only three days per week before the fire. Now, I usually work on patients only 10 days per month. Sometimes I feel a little guilty, but the feeling doesn't last long. It's like taking small vacations every single week, not to mention the actual long vacations I get to take at least once per quarter. Free time is certainly not a problem under our new system.

Making More Money – I don't like talking about actual dollar amounts, but it is true that under the Silicon Valley System, our overhead has never been lower and our profit margin never higher. I feel like one of the greatest things the system does for any practice is to rev up the motivational engine of the entire team while simultaneously slashing overhead. That adds up to a big win for everyone involved. Plus, the team gets to earn bonus money as a result of their hard work to make the practice better. It is an amazing thing to see.

In the following chapters I will share my vision with you. I hope it sparks a new hope in you that eventually will be kindled into a flame that lights the way to make your unique vision a reality.

I also hope it will make your biggest dreams come true—the way it has for me and my team.

CHAPTER ONE
TELL ME ABOUT YOUR DREAM PRACTICE

I have a big question for you.

Have you ever dreamed of having a practice that runs itself?

Picture this with me: You come into the office, look over the day's schedule, treat the patients, and then go home in time for a wonderful and relaxing dinner with your family. You are confident that all the stressful day-to-day details at the office are being handled by your team. Plus, your team members are steadily and happily working toward building you the practice of your dreams.

It's a nice dream, right?

There are dentists out there who are living a dream just like that, and they all have one big secret in common. Would you like to know what that secret is?

The one secret behind every truly successful practice is having enthusiastic and motivated dental team members who can make the doctor's vision of a dream practice come to life.

The only catch is that dental team members don't just wake up in the morning wanting to make the doctor's dreams a reality. They have to be inspired, and they need structure.

You might ask, "What's the simplest and most powerful way to inspire a dental team to behave like that?"

The answer is simple and can be revealed in one word, yet that word has been so abused over the years that it has almost become blasphemy among dentists.

This dental curse word represents a motivational tool that has the power to inspire and drive new heights of success for your practice. However, it also has the power to level and destroy teamwork and camaraderie, leaving a wake of destruction when it is misused.

You may think it sounds scary even to consider unleashing such a powerful force inside the entity that earns a living for your family. You may be the kind of dentist who would rather spend the rest of your career trudging to work and feeling secure in your misery.

If that describes you, then put down this book and go about your daily grind. You don't feel the need to see your practice reach its true potential, and that's fine. It's not for everyone.

But if you are brave enough to open Pandora's Box and witness what comes out, with hopes of harnessing the massive power waiting to be unleashed, then let's move forward.

So, what are these powerful, yet massively dangerous tools of practice growth that so many dentists avoid and despise?

Bonuses, of course.

I know what you're thinking. I already have a bonus or I tried that once or, even worse, I know somebody who had a bonus that blew up in his face (and not in a good way).

If you're looking for an argument, I'm not going to disagree. While I know that bonuses are the most powerful motivational tools available, they can be very dangerous. Sometimes offering your staff a bonus is like throwing gasoline on a fire (also not in a good way!).

The key to using bonuses effectively is to have the right system in place to contain them and harness their power. When you have the right system in place, you can motivate and reward your team without creating a monster bonus system that will eventually wreck your practice and make everyone in your office miserable. It is possible to craft a bonus system that is sustainable and perpetual, that lowers stress and overhead (they're related), all with a happy team of overachievers who can take you to the next level, building your practice to where you've always wanted it to be.

That's the aforementioned dream, right? It was definitely my dream, but I had to live through some nightmares before I achieved it.

You may be wondering why I am the guy to solve this problem for our profession. One reason would be experience, and by experience, I mean I've done just about everything wrong that you can imagine. Everything you can do wrong owning or managing a dental practice, I've done wrong. Luckily, I also have a history of good course corrections every time I realized the practice was headed in the wrong direction. Over time, my team and I found the things that absolutely worked, that laid the groundwork not only for our success but also for so many other practices with which we've had the honor to share our concepts and systems.

The only times we got close to making mistakes from which we couldn't recover were those times we got entangled with bad bonus systems. It's not just our practice that has experienced catastrophic effects from misguided employee incentives; our profession is plagued with many bonus systems that range from disastrous to nonsensical.

There are three popular bonus systems that are especially dangerous and damaging. I'm proud to say I have survived all of them at one point or another in my journey; however, I didn't escape without them leaving a few scars.

CHAPTER TWO
THE 3 DENTAL DEATH SPIRAL BONUSES DECODED

The big question in any dental practice is this: How do we motivate team members to achieve and maintain a great attitude every single day? Before we answer that question, let's look at how we *shouldn't* motivate them. This is an area where you will benefit greatly from my trial and error experimentation with those dangerous entities I call the death spiral bonus systems.

I've identified three of these practice-killing bonus systems: 1) bonus pool; 2) hourly above baseline; and 3) single statistic.

DEATH SPIRAL BONUS #1: BONUS POOL SYSTEM

The Promise of This Bonus: You will always keep your payroll overhead at a preset percentage, like 20% of collections. Your team will want to grow the practice because as the practice grows, their slice of the bonus pie grows, too.

Under a bonus pool system, all team members get a share of profits. As an example, let's say the practice needs to make $100,000 per month to break even. This month the practice brings in $120,000, and you've chosen to give 20% of the overage of $20,000 to your team. That comes to $400. If you have four team members, they each will get $100, five team members will get $80, and so on. The more team members you have, the lower the bonus for each person.

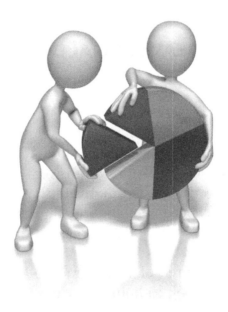

A bonus pool system won't work for long. Your team members will do just about anything to keep you from hiring new staff because new team members will further divide the bonus pie. You'll hear things like "We don't need anybody else. We've got this." When you do eventually need to hire more people, your team members will bicker about who's really doing most of the work. Since everyone gets the same amount, your team members who are pulling their weight will resent sharing the bonus with someone who they think is not working as hard. A bonus pool won't work forever. Eventually you will end up with a disgruntled staff.

Eventual Bad Result: Your practice will plateau because your team will fear the addition of more team members to split their piece of the bonus pie. New hires will get mistreated by veteran staff in a passive-aggressive attempt to convince you that the new people just don't fit in and aren't working out. Increased office stress is inevitable. Entire staff walkouts have happened.

DEATH SPIRAL BONUS #2: HOURLY ABOVE BASELINE

The Promise of This Bonus: You never have to give raises because your team's pay rises as the practice rises. They will want to grow the practice so their pay will increase.

Under an hourly above baseline system, the employees' wages are based on what the practice is making each month. The baseline is set when the employee is hired. When the practice's income goes up, the hourly wage goes up. Sounds great, right?

This system can actually work well for a short period of time because the original team members will work hard to grow the practice to make their pay go up. But at some point in time, the practice is going to slow down and/or you're going to need to hire more people. When you hire additional staff, the practice will have already grown so much that these new hires cannot earn a bonus that comes even close to the ones enjoyed by your longtime employees.

Of course, under the hourly above baseline system, your current employees would love for you to hire as many people as you can possibly afford. You'll hear things like "We need you to hire someone to do x, y, or z. We're swamped." Here is their thinking: A) more staff will grow the practice (and our bonus); and B) we can offload some of the work we're doing right now and get even more money for doing less work.

Here you have a recipe for disaster. Your new hires' bonuses will never catch up to the amount your long-term employees are making, so your newer employees will begin grumbling and morale will go down. Plus, in this model you can't outrun your growing overhead. You need to keep hiring more and more people, and as human nature kicks in, unhappy employees will be getting less and less done.

Eventual Bad Result: You will get less and less productivity from team members as they get more guaranteed money from the bonus. Your team will always try to get you to hire more people to spread out their workload. High overhead is inevitable, as is a very tired doctor with a sore back.

DEATH SPIRAL BONUS #3: SINGLE STATISTIC

The Promise of This Bonus: A few key statistics drive most of the revenue of the practice. Attaching one of these to a qualified staff member, like new patient acquisition, will make that staff person focus laser-like on growing that one key statistic. Then, as that statistic grows, the rising tide will lift the entire practice's growth.

A single statistic bonus is where you reward a person for accomplishing a single goal. This system can be fun—for a while. There was a time when I had a war room with the walls lined with statistic goals that our staff members had posted to keep themselves motivated. The problem with single-statistic bonuses is that they almost always favor the front office. For example, it's easy to quantify booking a goal number of appointments. It's harder to quantify clinical staff statistics. Dental assistants usually pitch in and help each other. It would be counterproductive to assign an assistant to a particular room to make it easier to quantity his or her work. Because it is easier to quantify statistics for the front office, eventually you will default to it, and those staff will get more of the bonus money. And even among your front office staff, if one person answers the phone more than the others, your other team members will resent that person.

The single statistic bonus can also lead to manipulation of the statistics, such as booking a large number of lower fee clients as new patients even though the practice may not be able to maintain profitability if the most profitable times are filled with these lower fee cases.

Like the other death spiral bonus systems, any benefit to the practice will be limited, and the bonus can actually reduce production and result in an unhappy staff.

Eventual Bad Result: One superstar will emerge and garner almost all of the bonus money. As your superstar's pay increases, resentment against that staff person and the entire bonus structure will ensue from the other team members. As the measured statistics eventually level out, your superstar's unhappiness coupled with the ongoing unhappiness of everyone else will cause the chosen metric to become neutered. A high office-misery index is inevitable.

HOW TO IDENTIFY A DEATH SPIRAL BONUS BEFORE IT'S TOO LATE

One of the things about these bonus systems that makes them so dangerous is the initial boost they give the practice. At first, my experience with one of these bonuses was great. We began producing three times the national average working only three days a week. Outwardly, all the signs of massive success were there, but the untold story is my overhead was about 70%. I was paying way too much for the production my practice generated, and I started to see that the bonus was slowly eating away at my practice. My staff had stopped seeing this extra money as a bonus for achieving a goal and more like a salary they deserved just for showing up for work every day.

Some of you reading this might be thinking that you don't really need to improve or motivate your team members. Maybe they are already great, even superstars in your eyes. If that's the case, congratulations. But what if something happens that shakes your world and shatters the practice you have worked so hard to build?

It happened to me, and the aftermath was the loss of not only my physical practice, but also more than 75 years of dental team experience.

HELP! I'M STUCK IN A BONUS!

So, what if you're currently stuck in one of the death spiral bonuses?

First of all, take a moment to breathe and consider your options. I would never recommend changing the way your team is compensated all at once. People get upset when you start tinkering with the way they are paid, especially when you talk about eliminating a bonus they've come to expect. There's a reason why I call them death spiral bonuses. They are tricky and hard to eliminate once you realize they are limiting your growth and making everyone in your practice unhappy.

But I have good news. The Silicon Valley Bonus System will fit in with any bonus you're currently using, and it is easily modified to wean staff members off a bad bonus into the full-time Silicon Valley Bonus System. The key is to ease into it. Don't rush in and make immediate changes to the way your team is used to being paid. Too much change too fast is scary. Eventually you will be able to ease out of your old bonus and use the power of the Silicon Valley Bonus to its fullest extent. Read on to learn how.

CHAPTER THREE
SILICON VALLEY MEETS DISNEY: LEARN HOW WALT DISNEY AND STEVE JOBS INSPIRED THE MOST AMAZING TEAM BONUS SYSTEM IN HISTORY

If it seems that dentistry and Silicon Valley are odd bedfellows, let me take you down the path that led me to develop this bonus system.

One hot summer Orlando day, I was visiting Disney World with my family, and we ducked into the Walt Disney museum to get out of the weather for a few minutes. As I toured the exhibits, I came upon one in particular that explained how Walt and his company had created a concept, revolutionary for its time, called storyboarding.

That's when the bells in my mind went off. It struck me that this concept fit hand in glove with a software creation concept developed in Silicon Valley that I had been reading about, called Scrum. I immediately knew that these two ideas combined would be a perfect solution for some of the implementation struggles we were having at my dental practice.

Dentistry has certainly seen benefits from Scrum already. Think about all the advances we have seen in software over the last couple of decades. Twenty years ago when we updated our dental software, it happened once per year, and it was on hard disk! Now we get updates almost weekly. That is the power of innovation, and the epicenter for that is Silicon Valley.

Home to Steve Jobs, Jeff Bezos, Mark Zuckerberg, and Google, Silicon Valley has produced some of the most amazing work environments in the history of the world, and all of it in our lifetime. We can learn a lot from these Silicon Valley entrepreneurs ... and Walt Disney.

You might be wondering about the link between Walt and Silicon Valley. It's a very intriguing story, and it involves another technology titan, Steve Jobs, and the decade he spent away from Apple.

WHAT DID STEVE JOBS KNOW ABOUT RUGBY AND DISNEY?

Before I share this interesting story about Steve Jobs, let me take a moment to address the elephant in the room. We are dentists. None of us is Steve Jobs (or Jeff Bezos or Mark Zuckerberg or the CEO of Google). Still, I'm sure all of us would love to have that amazing Silicon Valley success in our practice. There is a way we all can tap into that Silicon Valley magic, and it has everything to do with structuring a bonus system.

There are many reasons why any dentist might be reluctant to start a new bonus or modify an existing one, even if it has been proven to drive massive growth. Maybe you've been burned by using bonuses in your practice, perhaps you're nervous about the consequences of changing things, or it could be you're confused about all the small details. I get it. I've been there. But what I'm getting ready to tell you should remove a lot of the doubt that might be holding you back from creating the practice of your dreams.

Steve Jobs, in his second stint at Apple, did something amazing. He harnessed the power of Scrum, that exciting new concept that was making the rounds in Silicon Valley.

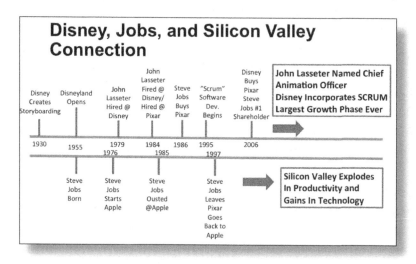

Scrum was a new way of implementing systems and creating software. It was named for the way a rugby team moves the ball down the field. I was shocked to learn that Steve Jobs combined Scrum with the storyboarding concept that Walt Disney created way back in 1930 and used this powerful combination to grow Apple into the biggest company in the world. Intrigued? So was I!

Before the Magic Kingdom and Cinderella's Castle, Walt Disney was a movie maker. His motion pictures were groundbreaking, and they built the Disney empire. He was talented at so many things, but above everything else, Disney was an innovator. He looked at the status quo and figured out how to make it better. Before Disney entered the film-making scene, people would write stories and make drawings, but they didn't know how to leverage the creative process.

Walt's team came up with the idea of tacking up the drawings for their animated movies and story concepts on the walls of his studio. His team members could walk around the room with their minds leaping from idea to idea, letting creativity flow. This way the artists and the storytellers discovered new directions and new paths to get to the end product in a fast-moving process. This process, of course, is the one we call storyboarding.

Back to Steve Jobs. You may remember that he started Apple in 1976. He got fired from Apple in 1985. After nine years with Apple, Jobs had plenty of money but nothing interesting to do with his wealth. He wanted to stay in the technology game, so he bought a company called Pixar. This is where the Steve Jobs-Disney connection comes in. Pixar was run by Disney-trained executives, including John Lasseter. Steve and John worked together at Pixar for over a decade, forming a strong friendship as well as a profitable partnership.

When Apple asked Steve Jobs to come back in 1997, it has been said that Steve told John he was willing to stay at Pixar out of loyalty to their friendship. I can only imagine that, being the great friend he was, John said, "Hey man, I think Apple's your calling." Steve Jobs went back to Apple, and the rest is history.

Apple's legendary business success exploded when Steve Jobs returned, applying his knowledge of innovative software coupled with the Disney creative concepts he had learned while at Pixar. It wasn't long before everyone in Silicon Valley started copying Apple, resulting in the largest productivity gains in technology in the history of the world. The statistics bear this out. When Steve went back to Apple in 1997, Apple stock was at $7 per share. As of this writing, a single share of Apple stock will set you back about $190, not including the previous splits.

An interesting side note to this story is that Disney bought Pixar in 2006, making Steve Jobs its number one shareholder. Steve's influence likely resulted in John Lasseter being named chief animation officer. Friendship is a beautiful thing, and profitable, too. Disney stock soared, from $20 in 2006 to more than $100 currently.

Today, if you want to work in management for Disney, you need to be proficient in the Scrum software concept. Clearly this concept has been a winner in Silicon Valley, and it's working for Disney, too. The good news is you can make it work for your practice, especially when you learn how to combine it with Disney's storyboarding technique.

Stick with me on this, and I will spell out exactly how you can use the Scrum and storyboarding concepts in your practice. When you apply these concepts correctly, you'll be a happy, stress-free doctor with an enthusiastic and motivated team. My goal is to help every dentist reading this book to have the staff of their dreams. I'm talking about having that happy, motivated team that makes our lives easier, not harder. Plus, you can have your dream staff without falling victim to one of those death spiral bonuses that have wrecked so many practices. If you have had a bad experience with a bonus in the past, I want to convince you that not all bonuses are evil—but only if you apply them using a solid strategy that considers all the long-term ramifications that so many practice owners fail to acknowledge. Obviously, bonuses are not the answer by themselves. If they were, every dentist and small business owner would employ them at all times. Bonuses have a bad name for a reason. Many times an ill-thought-out bonus system wreaks havoc on the office's overhead and tranquility. But it doesn't have to be that way. Any good bonus plan needs the right system supporting it, and I've found this support in the Silicon Valley Bonus System, something never heard of in dentistry before. Read to the end, and I'll give you a step-by-step cookbook on how to start using the Silicon Valley Bonus System in your practice right away. In the meantime, here's a quick look at the structure of the Silicon Valley Bonus:

The Silicon Valley Bonus System has three important components: the doctor, the team members, and the Scrum master, who we'll refer to as the Practice Promoter to avoid the confusion of comparing a true technology-based Scrum master to one who administers the Silicon Valley Bonus in a dental practice.

❑ The doctor provides the vision.
❑ Each team member selects or is assigned bite-sized pieces of that vision to implement.
❑ The Practice Promoter keeps the team headed in the right direction, ensuring that tasks are completed by happy team members.

Completed Tasks + Happy Team Members =
A Happy Doctor!

I explained the term *Scrum* earlier in this chapter. To review, it is a technique that rugby players use to move the ball down the field. In the business world, it is a technique that keeps the vision of a business moving forward. The beauty of using Scrum in a dental practice is that it allows your team members to choose the tasks they want to complete. In the engineering world, this would be called a pull system instead of a push system.

In a push system, things get pushed down a conveyor belt and the workers are expected to keep up. Think about Lucy and Ethel trying to package chocolates in that famous episode of *I Love Lucy*, and you get the idea. It's a mess!

Scrum is a pull system, which is more organized and people driven. In a pull system, people are identified to do specific things coming down the conveyor belt. Each person goes to the conveyor belt, takes the item off the belt, and takes it to completion. No one has "chocolates" flying at them faster than they can package (or eat) them.

Within the dental practice, we refer to the Scrum master as the Practice Promoter. The Practice Promoter ensures the completion of individual tasks by helping to solve problems and challenges as they arise. The doctor leaves the day-to-day practice details in the hands of the Practice Promoter. There's no need to micromanage. Your vision moves forward because happy team members understand the vision and have a series of small tasks to complete, all under the watchful eye of the Practice Promoter.

When you learn how to implement the Silicon Valley Bonus System, you'll be amazed by how little time it takes away from the dental chair or your free time. I call myself the Lunch Hour CEO because I was able to sit down with my team for about an hour over lunch—one time—to hammer out the vision we wanted for our practice. That was two years ago. Since then, I've spent about 10 minutes per week working on my part of the Silicon Valley Bonus System. It's the best, most fun 10 minutes I spend each week! More on that later in the book.

Once you implement the Silicon Valley Bonus System, your team becomes the real leader of the practice. When your employees understand your vision and have the motivation to make it a reality, they take over so you can focus on the patients while your team focuses on keeping the practice running smoothly. The best part of this bonus system is that it's not based on money.

What do I mean by that? Most of the death spiral bonuses are based on how much money the practice makes, either in production or collections. The team members are rewarded accordingly and enriched as the practice grows, but they suffer when the practice suffers.

It sounds good in theory; however, remember that you don't have the right to keep any staff members working at your practice against their will, and there will always be cycles in any business. I have personally seen all the most popular bonuses do irreparable harm to practices, including the loss of patients, staff members, and even early retirements due to stress. In truth, production and collections are terrible benchmarks of practice health, and in many circumstances become arbitrary over time.

1. Arbitrary money measurements destroy practices.
2. Money-based bonuses can quickly become monster bonuses.
3. Money-based bonuses will eventually cause strife.

Sure, money-based bonuses can quickly drive up your numbers, but it will be temporary. Like a cocaine high, it is very likely that soon those numbers are going to go back down. If you are paying a consultant that teaches you a specific money-based bonus, isn't it ironic that it's usually shortly after that consultant gets paid that your numbers start to drop? Money-based bonuses are also well known for causing dissension among staff members, and they can even influence the dentist's judgment on whether or not to take a case when the team needs a little more production to make a bonus milestone. The bottom line is this: Money-based bonuses become monster bonuses that will drag your practice down if you let them hang around too long.

SILICON VALLEY BONUSES OFFER THESE THREE BIG BENEFITS:

1. Your team can be motivated to earn bonus money in a way that sustainably grows the practice and cannot lose effectiveness over time. This usually lets you fire expensive consultants and ditch those monster bonuses.

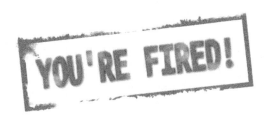

You, the doctor, can turn virtually every burdensome task you hate over to your team and they will solve the problems (and be happy about it!).

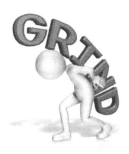

2. This bonus opens the door to the possibility of more time off for you, the doctor, with no decrease in production, because of the good work of your team.

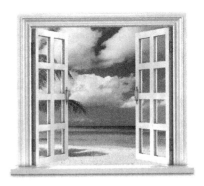

You may think your team is happy making whatever you pay them now, whether it's a salary or an hourly wage. That's a myth. Here's the truth:

*There is ALWAYS another level of achievement your
team members could reach IF they had the proper
motivation and felt validated for their efforts.*

THE THREE V'S YOU NEED TO GROW

To grow your practice, you need the Three V's: Vision, Vehicle,
and Validation. Master the Three V's, and your team members
will be motivated, they will take ownership of your practice
growth, and you will no longer have to deal with menial tasks
you hate. I cover each V in detail in the following chapters.

CHAPTER FOUR
JOB #1: CREATE A VISION FOR YOUR PRACTICE

The very first thing that must be done to make this a reality is for you, the doctor, to become crystal clear about the direction you want to pursue with your practice. Every dentist and every practice is different. No one can decide what kind of practice will make you happiest. Take all the time you need to imagine this. There is a process that I sometimes take dentists through when they take my courses called the Core Beliefs Exercise. In that exercise, I have them imagine what it would be like if they lived their life to the fullest with no consequences. Where would they live? What would they eat? Where would they work? What kind of dentistry would they do? On what kind of patients? You get the idea. I'm trying to dig deeply into their true desires. Once we know what that looks like, we can start building the closest resemblance of that in reality. It's a beautiful exercise and one I did for myself years ago with great success.

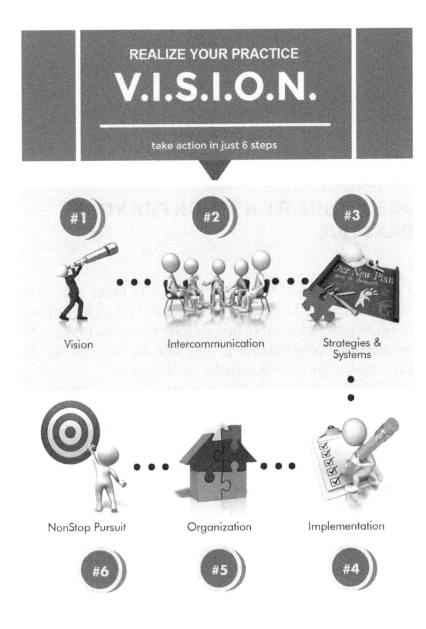

Once the doctor's vision is set, it is time to find a helper. The doctor cannot be expected to carry out all the demands of making that vision come true. If that were required, 99% of dentists would practice in a very unfulfilling way. The doctor needs another person in the trenches with them every day who can take the majority of the management burdens off them so they can focus on taking great care of their patients and help the practice grow that way.

The perfect person to help the doctor in this way is a person I call the Practice Promoter. We will discuss their job description in detail in a later chapter, but suffice it to say that they are the second most important person in the practice when it comes to making the doctor's vision of the practice come true.

Naming the Practice Promoter is the second and last task we will ask the doctor to perform to make the Silicon Valley Bonus System a reality.

After the Practice Promoter is named, the doctor needs to make sure that they are well informed about what will be expected of them and share the practice vision with them. After a nice long meeting about expectations and any clarifications the Practice Promoter might need, it's time to take the vision to the rest of the team. Sitting down with your team to develop a shared vision is the first step toward implementing the Silicon Valley Bonus System. If you are going to ask your team members to make your life better by removing the bulk of your management burdens, they need to have an active voice in defining that practice vision.

Sitting down with your team to develop a shared vision is the first step toward implementing the Silicon Valley Bonus System. If you are going to ask your team members to make your life better by removing the bulk of your management burdens, they need to have an active voice in defining that practice vision.

Here's what I suggest. Call a lunch hour meeting and maybe even make it an hour and a half. This could be the most important hour and a half of planning you ever do. During your meeting, follow this six-step V.I.S.I.O.N. process:

1. Define your practice **Vision** by asking your team members what kind of workday would be their idea of the most amazing practice day possible. Don't limit their imagination at this point by throwing up artificial barriers. If they say they would like to see only clear braces patients and have daily two-hour lunches, allow that train of thought to move forward even if you think it is out of the realm of re-alistic possibility. Once everyone has had a chance to describe their idea of a perfect day, you can share your idea of what a perfect day looks like to you.

2. Next, almost in the same way that Congress goes to committee to hammer out a final bill between the House and the Senate, you need to facilitate **In-tercommunication**. Discuss what is and is not feasible at this exact juncture. You may very well discover that your team will become more moti-vated as they are allowed a voice in the overall di-rection of the practice, and that should make your job moving forward much easier. At the end of the intercommunication session, you should have a first draft of your practice vision.

MY BIG RED BOOK

Here is a photo of Griffin Dental's Big Red Book. This book holds all of my systems, job descriptions, marketing campaigns, projects, and referral programs, basically everything in my practice. This book included everything I needed to start over when my

practice burned down in 2013. While it's not a substitute for using an online computer backup service (which I was very thankful to have), I was thrilled to find this book basically intact after the fire.

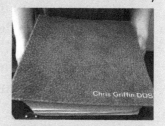

Chris Griffin DDS

I highly recommend you have one of these hard copy books in your practice. The creation of this book itself will almost guarantee a huge increase in productivity. If disaster were to strike you, it could save you hundreds of thousands of dollars by keeping your practice held together until you can get caught up.

3. Next, you need to begin the process of defining and developing **Strategies** that will lead to the systems that will make your shared vision come true. You should leave this meeting with everyone on the same page and receptive to the changes you are going to install that will make everyone's lives better in the long run.

4. After you and your leadership team have gotten the basic two or three beginning systems in the blueprint phase that you would like to become status quo in the practice, **Implement** them. Implementation is sometimes considered a dirty word in dentistry because all dentists know how hard it is to change. Resistance to change is universal. It not only applies to the team, but also to the dentist. But we all know that movement toward our goals

isn't possible without change, so implementation is the key. I like to have a quick meeting with my leadership team to get everyone on the same page as to the exact steps we will need to take in order to make our vision in a particular area happen. Then I usually let my team leaders do the implementation. Of course, I like to be there whenever questions arise so we can keep revising our systems blueprint to continue moving in the right direction.

5. Once our systems are running smoothly, whether that takes a couple of weeks or a couple of months, we memorialize our **Organization** by writing down all the steps and systems it took to create our new and improved working environment. I like to keep a hard copy of all of our systems in a three-ring binder, but you can also do this on a computer. No matter which you use, be sure to have backups! As I learned in my fire, some things can never be recovered if lost, and you certainly don't want to lose a book of the systems that are helping you realize your dream practice. This book is an amazing resource for review, and it's also a great training resource for new hires. Once systems are written down, you can always revisit and revise them. This is more of a living document than a permanent set of office commandments.

6. Finally, I suggest you continually repeat this process. I call this **Nonstop pursuit**, and it is the last piece of the puzzle. You should never stop pursuing your goals and dreams. Plus, if your team helped

you create the vision of your practice and you are all pursuing that goal together, it exponentially increases the chance your team members will take ownership of the new vision.

With your vision in place, your next step is to give your team a vehicle to take them to that vision. It's the topic of our next chapter.

CHAPTER FIVE
GIVE YOUR TEAM A VEHICLE TO ACHIEVE YOUR SHARED VISION

The six-step V.I.S.I.O.N. process takes care of everyone knowing the direction in which they need to drive the practice, but they still need a vehicle that provides them motivation on a daily or weekly basis. Creating an environment of success is part of that, but you also need specific tools to help create the new environment. The success vehicle in our practice is our Silicon Valley Bonus Board. This is a centrally located board that tracks all the ongoing projects that are going on in the practice at any given time.

All those systems and blueprints that you created in the V.I.S.I.O.N. process can and should be broken up into bite-sized tasks. In our office we take one hour per week away from treating patients to work on our Silicon Valley Bonus Board. Here's the process we use:

Either I or my leadership team is continually making lists of new tasks that need to be accomplished in the practice. For example, if we are going to design a new marketing campaign to target students at our local college, we need someone to: 1) figure out a good offer that might attract those students; 2) draw up a mockup of a marketing piece; 3) work with a printer to get the marketing brochure, flyer, or postcard printed to our specs; and 4) deliver the pieces to the prospective new patients in whatever way we choose. Those four distinct tasks can be placed on our Bonus Board and worked on during our weekly implementation hour by any members of our team who would like to choose them. The beauty of this system is that all of our team members can pick and choose whichever tasks appeal to them during this weekly hour. When they pick the task, they own it, and that makes all the difference in their effort levels and motivation.

OLD MODEL: REACTIVE

The old model of running a practice is reactive. When bad things happen to the doctor, the doctor gets upset and tells someone, such as the office manager, that the bad thing needs to be fixed. The employee doesn't know exactly what to do, and either does something the doctor doesn't like or sets aside the problem and hopes the subject never comes up again. The doctor either forgets about it until something bad happens again, or he or she gets mad and decides to do it him or herself—always a bad idea. The old model causes stress, anger, frustration, and doubt.

NEW MODEL: PROACTIVE

The model I outline in this book is proactive. It is a structured system with the vehicle in place to deal with completing tasks as they come up.

Once you have your vision and your vehicle in place, you need to provide validation to your team members so they know you recognize and appreciate their contributions to the success of the practice.

CHAPTER SIX
VALIDATION KEEPS THE VISION GOING

Your team members need you to recognize the efforts they are making to build your practice. This is where the Silicon Valley Bonus comes in.

THE POWER OF THE BONUS HOUR

We developed our validation bonus system after studying the ways that some of the most successful companies in Silicon Valley managed and rewarded their teams as they grew into giants of the industry. These companies still use boards just like the Silicon Valley Bonus Board I have been describing. In our case, we attach a dollar value to each of the bite-sized tasks that are placed on the board. When the team comes together for our "bonus hour" retrospective session each week, I validate their efforts and recognize their success. As they are working to make the practice stronger and moving toward our shared vision, they are also earning bonus money.

As I have discussed throughout this book, bonuses have a checkered past in our profession. I am not a proponent of overtly money-based bonuses that can create all kinds of trouble for your practice if they are not closely monitored. The Silicon Valley Bonuses I use in my practice are one-time payments that reward my team members for a job well done on each particular task.

You can be very conservative or very generous with your payouts, but as you write each team member an actual check for his or her efforts to make the practice better, you are validating that person as a valuable member of your team. This will pay you dividends that will take you to your ultimate goal much faster, and probably create a much better working environment along the way.

YOU HAVE TO SEE IT TO BELIEVE IT

Almost no dentist spends time working *on* the practice. They certainly spend time working *in* the practice. Most days, dentists are bombarded with questions and problems the second they step foot inside the door of the office. Then, as the daily grind of patient and staff issues wears them down, most only want to escape at the end of the day and find some respite at home or some other place far away from all the chaos.

The top practices seem to find a way to structure time during every day or week for the dental team to train and to grow the practice.

Those practices experience a phenomenon where the dividends from the efforts of team members during the "magic" bonus hour or hours exponentially surpass what we would typically expect from the amount of time spent.

Not to mention the fact that every time I have seen a dental practice take just one hour per week to work *on* the practice with a system like the Silicon Valley Bonus System, the practice's production has either remained the same or has gone up.

Sometimes the production goes way up.

If you implement the Three V's in your practice, you will be turning over some of the office leadership to your team. I know that relinquishing practice responsibilities can feel strange. It's in your nature to be the driver. That's what has made you successful so far. I just ask you to consider how great it would feel to be the hero to your patients, but not have to carry around all the worries and concerns of day-to-day practice operations.

The question is, are you brave enough to do what it takes to make this happen?

I suppose you just have to see it to believe it.

How is that possible with fewer patient treatment hours?

Maybe it's a paradox or maybe the problems that get solved and the creative ideas that spring from the mastermind created during these bonus sessions make the practice so efficient during the rest of the work week that production must go up.

This is one of those concepts that you must experience first-hand to truly believe. So, have some courage and take that leap of faith! Let me encourage you from my own experience:

I have never seen a practice go from 40 patient hours to 39 and go down in production.

I have never seen a practice go from 36 hours to 35 and go down.

I have never seen a practice go from 30 hours to 29 and go down.

I have seen doctors and team members become happier and more energetic, and practices become more profitable when patient hours decrease.

DON'T FORGET YOUR FREE BONUS TRAINING WEBINAR

Register for your bonus training that goes with this book by going to **www.SiliconValleyBonus.com** On this training, you will learn:

- How to **identify a Death Spiral Bonus** before it makes everyone miserable and kills your team unity

- How to apply the Silicon Valley System to your Practice in a way that could <u>double your practice and make your team love you for it!</u>

- You can **stop spending THOUSANDS each year with big marketing companies and slick consultants** who try to convince you that your results are better than they actually are.

- This is THE MISSING PIECE of the training for Implants, CEREC, Ortho, or any other highly advanced skills you have acquired. I <u>don't even think you should do those trainings until you learn this protocol.</u>

- This is THE answer for the age-old problem of doctor›s not having enough time to manage their team. **The Silicon Valley Secret will turn you into a Lunch Hour CEO** (and it won›t even take nearly the whole hour.)

- Once Your team starts seeing how this makes the practice better, THEY WILL LOVE YOU FOR IT!

Go to **www.SiliconValleyBonus.com** and sign up today

CHAPTER SEVEN
DON'T LET FEAR HOLD YOU BACK

One of the big myths is that you have to work more hours to make more money, right? The truth is almost no dentists spend any time working on their practice to begin with, they just don't. They go in, they get pummeled by problems, they are hammered by their staff, they treat patients (who many dentists view as problems themselves), and they drag themselves home at the end of the day to collapse and forget about their practice while they dream of a better life.

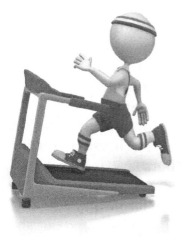

I've always heard that it's every dentist's dream is to do something else, meaning something outside of dentistry. Well, that's very sad; it shouldn't be that way. If dentists were brave enough to take away an hour a week from treating patients to work on their practice, they would see that they could probably do more production, working fewer hours, if they only had a better system in place.

The Silicon Valley Bonus System is that system.

If there's one thing I am confident about, it's the fact that I have worked toward the goal of working less and making more to create a better lifestyle during my entire career. I know a thing or two about how to cut back hours and still profitably grow a practice.

I always believed that more time spent at the office didn't necessarily equate to more money. In 2005, we started trimming full or half days off our work week every few months. Every time we took an extra day off from seeing patients each week, I was scared, but the practice numbers always went up. When we went from four days a week to three days a week in 2008, the practice actually went up $250,000!

Looking back, I clearly remember the day I made the decision to go to three patient days per week. I had been removing weeds from a watermelon patch on my farm on a Friday. It was considerably hot that day, and I was bemoaning the fact that I had to rush to finish because I needed to go home to get ready for a family function with my kids. If only I had Thursdays off from the practice, I could farm on Thursdays and Fridays, leaving plenty of time for family outings on the weekends. I wanted it all. I wanted to have time for my practice, my family, and even myself. That day I decided to go out six months into the future, so as not to hinder any hygiene patients who had already scheduled their appointments, and cross out every Thursday on my practice calendar.

I won't lie to you. After I made the decision, I was still scared to death. It was only logical that the practice would shrink since we were cutting our work week by 25%. So, during the six-month period leading up to my three-days-per-week leap of faith, we worked hard to install as many practice systems as possible, primarily focusing on clinical efficiency and new patient experiences.

It is no coincidence that when we put that much effort into our practice systems that the practice grew. There was nothing magical about going to three days per week; the practice grew because we had our systems in order. And our systems were in order because we had an implementation system to ensure they actually were installed into the practice, the Silicon Valley Bonus System.

I'VE BEEN THERE. I'VE DONE THAT.

Don't think I am preaching to you from an ivory tower. I've done a lot of things wrong along the way. I've used all of the death spiral bonuses at one time or another. I had a war room covered in more than 100 pieces of graph paper that charted goals we never accomplished. I have way overpaid for what I thought were superstars on my staff. I even placed earning caps on my best team members, trying to protect the worst team members! (That was an especially idiotic move.) One year I had 1,400 hours of meetings, which were really just gripe sessions, at the recommendation of one of those high-dollar consultants (which I hope you can fire after you learn the Silicon Valley Bonus System). I tried to be fair and pay everyone equally for the accomplishments of just a few superstars. I assumed all of my team members had the best interest of the practice in mind over their own interests. Are you kidding me?

ALONG THE WAY I DID GET A FEW THINGS RIGHT.

All those mistakes illustrate the one truth I learned after that fire burned down my practice in 2013. I have learned that you can't fight human nature, but you can harness it. The Silicon Valley Bonus System harnesses human nature better than any incentive plan I have ever seen.

Here's how all this came about. A while back I discovered the power of having team members take on bite-sized tasks instead of just proclaiming that an impossibly difficult change needed to be made. That early iteration worked relatively well at times, but it was rudderless. It didn't have a vision, and it lacked the spark of motivation that you absolutely need for this system to work. It didn't have validation. When I added the vision by going through the V.I.S.I.O.N. exercise, things finally started to go in the right direction. Then I added validation—it was like throwing gasoline on a fire. (It was nice to experience fire in a good way!) The system took off like a rocket ship; my team members started taking real ownership of not only their jobs, but also the growth and health of the practice. As they started to get it, I could almost feel the weight of the world lifted off my shoulders. Imagine how good it feels not to be stressed out and to be able to focus on the patients without worrying about the day-to-day grind that most dentists dread.

Imagine being able to see at a glance that your team is diligently working through tasks every day to make the practice better. Imagine never having to give someone a raise again if you don't want to. The Silicon Valley Bonus System keeps your team happy and engaged and your overhead low. Your overhead stops going up and even starts dropping due to the increased practice effectiveness, even as your team members feel validated with bonus monies for their efforts. Because it's not based on money measurements, the bonus system is 100% sustainable and perpetual as long as you continue to provide the vision for your practice. Who wouldn't want to do this?

LOOK WHO DOESN'T WANT YOU TO LEARN ABOUT THIS SYSTEM.

While I can't think of a dentist who wouldn't benefit from using the Silicon Valley Bonus System, there are a few entities that would prefer we dentists continue business as usual, relying on those death spiral bonus systems that work for a while but then drag us down, making us work harder to make less money.

Expensive consultants don't want you to learn about the Silicon Valley Bonus System. Why? Because it reveals the truth about them. Expensive consultants are not helping you do what needs to be done to be successful in your practice. This makes these consultants worse than useless.

Corporate dentistry is either owned by outside entities or has advisors from places like Silicon Valley. They already understand the Silicon Valley system, and they are using it against you. They certainly don't want to let you in on the secret!

Insurance companies would love for the majority of our profession to remain bogged down and stressed out so our practices aren't effective at treating their clients' dental needs. That way they don't have to write checks to us.

Have I made my case? Are you ready for the step-by-step cookbook for implementing the Silicon Valley Bonus System in your practice? Just turn the page!

CHAPTER EIGHT

THE SILICON VALLEY BONUS SYSTEM COOKBOOK
YOUR RECIPE FOR SUCCESS

You can implement the Silicon Valley Bonus System in six easy steps. Here they are:

STEP #1:

Develop and define your unique practice vision using the V.I.S.I.O.N. process.

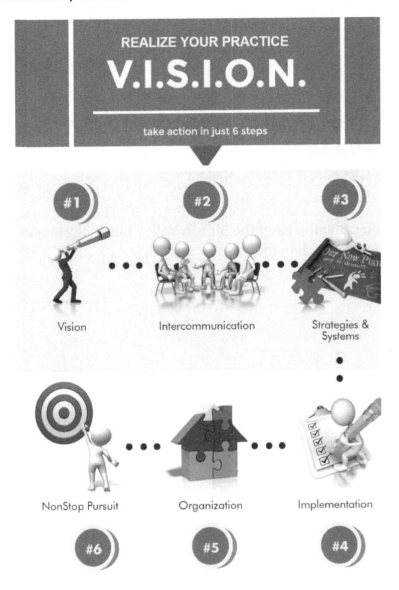

STEP #2:

Break down the vision into tasks needed to implement the vision and allow team members to choose which tasks they would like to complete.

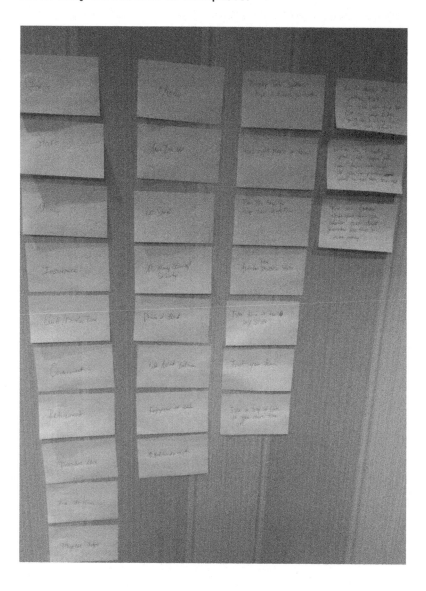

STEP #3:

Organize tasks using a Silicon Valley Bonus Board. The headers on the board should be ToDo, Designated Ready, Doing with a Deadline, and Done" You can use simple sticky notes like we do in our practice, or you may choose to use software, like Trello, to create a virtual board. Note: I highly recommend using a physical board for your practice at least in the beginning so you and your team can tap into the power of Visual Learning and Accountability. It is impossible to ignore an impending deadline when you have to walk past the physical board every day.

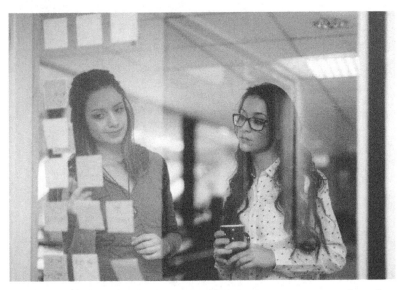

Versions of Silicon Valley Boards are found in top companies of all sizes all across the country

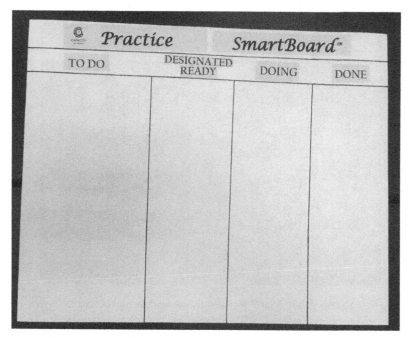

Blank simple Silicon Valley Bonus Board made from poster

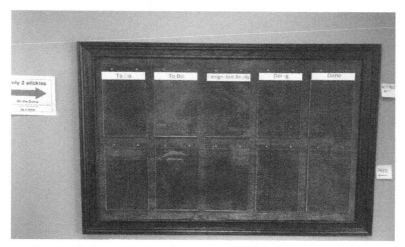

Blank Silicon Valley Bonus System Board at Dr. Griffin's office

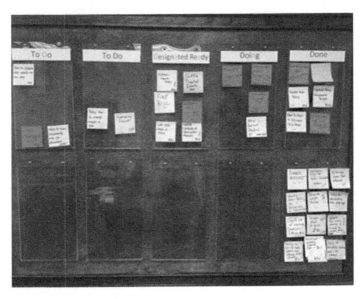

Silicon Valley Board during normal workweek in progress

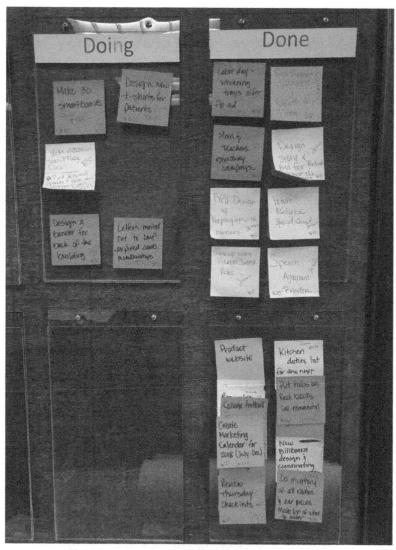

Up close look at ToDo tasks on Silicon Valley Bonus Board

STEP #4:

Name a Practice Promoter to act as Scrum master. Your Practice Promoter is very important. This person will ask the team members who own each task three questions during the weekly bonus hour/retrospective session. He or she should be an encourager and a problem-solver above all else. This person can take on tasks, but usually doesn't.

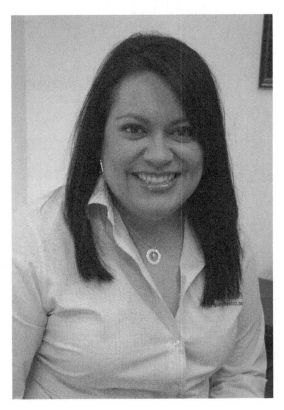

Lupita is our amazing Practice Promoter here at Griffin Dental and also coaches other offices on how to develop and train their own Practice Promoters.

STEP #5:

Have a weekly bonus hour/retrospective session. Take the first few minutes to hand out bonus checks for completed tasks. Quickly review the completed tasks. Ask for any questions from the team, and then you, the doctor, can leave the meeting. You should be able to accomplish this in about 10 minutes. Be sure to document completed tasks in something like my Big Red Book as a ready reference if something gets off track.

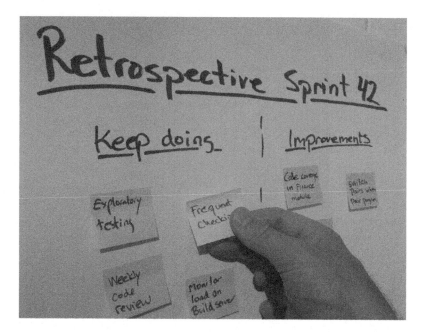

STEP #6:

Pursue your V.I.S.I.O.N. nonstop. If you as the doctor provide the vision, enable your staff members by providing the vehicle to pursue it, and motivate your people by providing validation, the Silicon Valley Bonus System will continue to grow your practice.

What took me 10 years to get right could literally take you only 10 days to get started and begin seeing results.

Silicon Valley Real Life Cookbook Examples

Here are some real-world examples of big projects that have been broken down into ToDos for the Silicon Valley Bonus Board

Project – Create Your First Facebook Ad

ToDos:

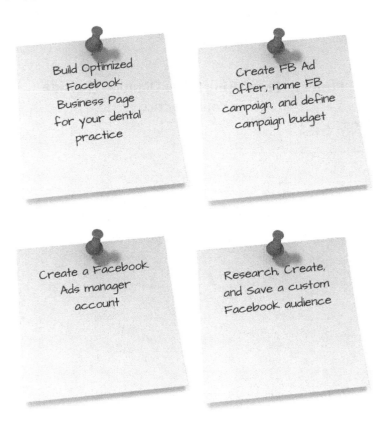

Build Optimized Facebook Business Page for your dental practice

Create FB Ad offer, name FB campaign, and define campaign budget

Create a Facebook Ads manager account

Research, Create, and Save a custom Facebook audience

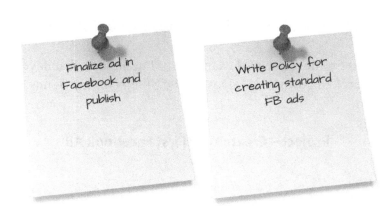

Project – Start Using Silver Diamine Fluoride in Your Practice

ToDos:

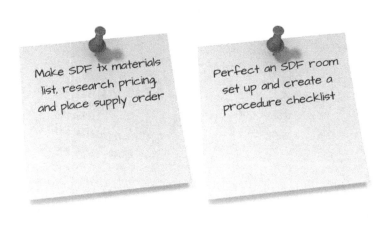

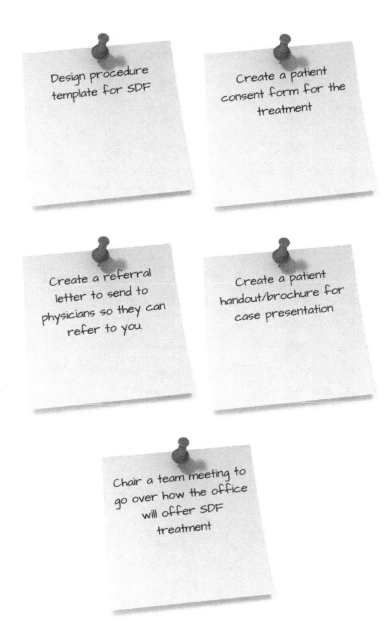

Design procedure template for SDF

Create a patient consent form for the treatment

Create a referral letter to send to physicians so they can refer to you.

Create a patient handout/brochure for case presentation

Chair a team meeting to go over how the office will offer SDF treatment

Project – Write and Send an End of the Year Marketing Letter to Patients

ToDos:

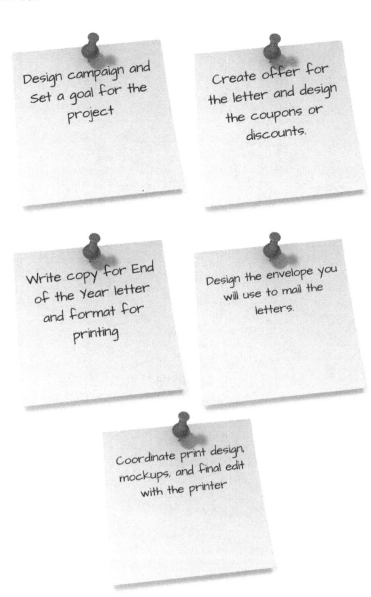

Design campaign and Set a goal for the project

Create offer for the letter and design the coupons or discounts.

Write copy for End of the Year letter and format for printing

Design the envelope you will use to mail the letters.

Coordinate print design, mockups, and final edit with the printer

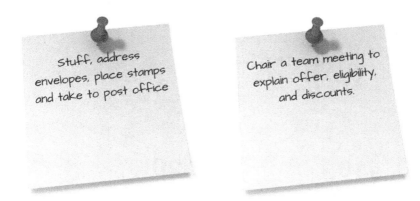

Now, here are those same ToDos ready to be moved to the designated ready column with an assigned dollar value.

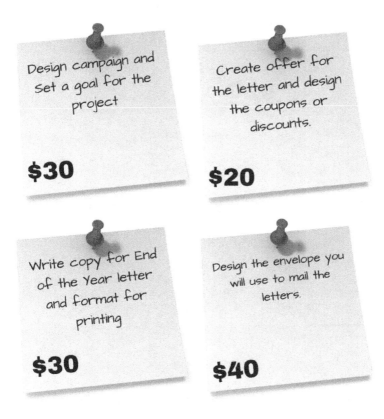

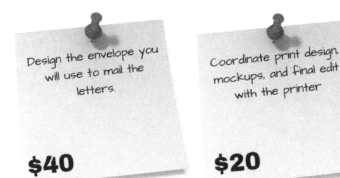

Design the envelope you will use to mail the letters.

$40

Coordinate print design, mockups, and final edit with the printer

$20

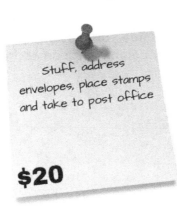

Stuff, address envelopes, place stamps and take to post office

$20

Here are those ToDos assigned to team members with deadlines as they are moved into the Doing with Deadline column.

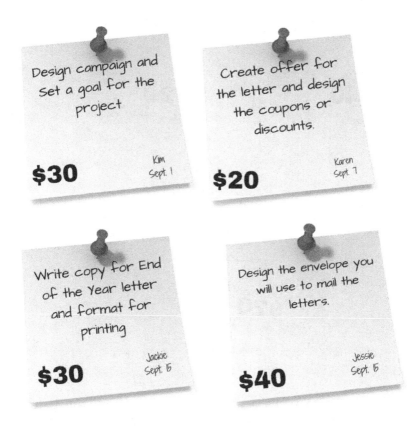

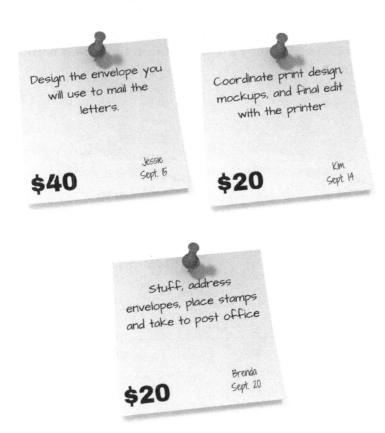

As these ToDo tasks are finished, they are taken to the Practice Promoter to approve and verify that they have truly been completed and then placed into the Done column until the next Retrospective meeting so the bonus money can be distributed and the team member can be recognized for their efforts.

CHAPTER NINE
WHY EVERYONE NEEDS A PRACTICE PROMOTER

Everyone already has a practice promoter. They are the person who is constantly juggling all the important and urgent projects in the practice. They are the ones who truly care if the practice fails or succeeds. They are always thinking of ways to help grow the practice. If they slow down the practice slows down. If they get distracted, the practice goes into a slump. When they are focused and on point, but practice is almost unstoppable.

If you don't know who your Practice Promoter is, then it is you. If you are thinking that you didn't realize that the job of Practice Promoter was that important, I am hoping you take this book seriously and implement the Silicon Valley Bonus System tomorrow because naming a Practice Promoter to help you implement this amazing piece of technology into your practice should be first on your agenda.

Let me take you back to a time in our practice before we instituted the Silicon Valley Bonus System. We were struggling with implementing the things that I knew could make a huge difference in our practice.

I truly believe that having the ability to add new ideas, procedures, and systems to your dental office is the one thing that will keep you afloat during tough times and explode with growth during good economic times. That means that to be effective, a dental practice needs to constantly be evolving. In turn, that means that the team needs to be implementing new ideas monthly if not weekly.

In my own practice, I didn't see how this was going to be possible without some big changes.

My staff was telling me that they were already maxed out already. If I suggested we learn a new technique or system, they would say that they needed more people and more time to be able to do what I wanted done.

I had a decision to make. I could either take their word for it and hire more people, further making my overhead a true headache, or I could try to find a way to utilize our time in the office better that we were currently.

I decided that I had to make some serious changes to our workweek, but I ran into roadblocks.

The staff was very hard to get on board.
They didn't like the idea of changing at all.

We had to come up with a way to get the staff on board, because the key to a dream practice lies with them. Without the staff on the dentist's side, all efforts will be in vain. We finally hit a home run when we discovered a way to get the staff all on the same page with me using the Silicon Valley System.

This system which utilized the services of a very special team member called a Practice Promoter very much benefit the team. However, the very best benefits are for the doctor. The doctor gets the benefits of having a happy, motivated staff, and they really don't have to do all that much to get this system going.

All We Ask the Doctor to Do is ONE Thing!

The doctor only must come up with the vision of the practice, that's it. Then, they can hand off the implementation of the system to the second most important team member in the office, the Practice Promoter.

The Practice Promoter gives you:

❑ Freedom and comfort to KNOW that your staff is being productive and growing.
❑ Someone who actually cares if the team is continually striving to reach your practice goals.
❑ A built-in buffer between you and any challenges or confusion about new ideas and new implementations in the practice.
❑ Someone in the office to share in your ownership mentality.
❑ The list goes on and on.....

Our definition of a Practice Promoter

They are a highly-trained set of eyes and ears in a dental practice that can become a surrogate of the doctor in management, training, motivation, and performance of the other team members at that dental practice.

They should understand the vision of the practice. They must be well-respected, organized, have a well-rounded skill set, work well with others, be sincere, have the ability to problem solve, and they also must be outstanding encouragers to the rest of the team. They also must give honest feedback to their people. The must be someone who can sit with team members, look them in the eye, ask them good questions, and give them honest feedback. They must be able to measure results. They must be able to not only measure them, but understand what it means when they measure them. The Practice Promoter is NOT a supervisor or a micromanager. They are not a snitch. They don't run to the doctor every time another team member goes astray. They are also not to lord over the other teammates as if they have special privileges in the practice. They are truly to become servants to not only the practice goals, but also to the other staff members they are helping along the way. Think of them as another set of eyes and ears for the doctor who is also on the side of the employees. They are a very unique combination indeed.

There are 8 basic traits needed for any Practice Promoter to succeed. Let's go over them one by one.

8 Practice Promoter Traits

Trait #1 - Encourager
- First and foremost, the Practice Promoter needs to build team morale and end intra-office rivalries forever by proper interactions with the team. The team leader must become a cheerleader. There is no way around it. Attitude and enthusiasm are a must, not only for the Practice Promoter, but for the whole team if the team is going to achieve the vision of the doctor.

Trait #2 – Time Manager

❏ The Practice Promoter must maximize accomplishment during periods of Bonus Time in the practice. The Practice Promoter is the person who the rest of the team will look towards to keep projects and task moving forward toward their deadlines. The Practice Promoter must run effec-tive Silicon Valley Bonus Time with or without the doctor. This time is important for the staff and the practice. To effectively manage the Bonus Board they must have great communication skills.

Trait #3 – Project Manager

❏ The Practice Promoter must develop realistic but challenging projects for the practice that align with the doctor's vision with realistic deadlines. The doctor is going to give the visionary guidance, but it is up to the team and the Practice Promoter to get down on the ground level and develop realistic and challenging projects and tasks for the team. The Practice Promoter must create new projects continually that promote good experiences for the patients. Those are going to lead to direct patient referrals. Those are the juice or the fuel that makes the practice go. Direct patient referrals are so much more powerful than advertising patients. They are worth more to the practice. They don't cost as much to get, and they are worth more in the long run. The team leader must uncover new ways to make the patients feel special.

Trait #4 - Empathizer

❏ The Practice Promoter needs to have an understand-ing when to push the team and when to let off the gas a bit. When things get strained, the staff gets stressed. When the staff gets stressed, they can handle that for a while, but not forever. If the team feels prolonged periods of stress, bad things will happen. You will have bad performances by your team. You will have high-tension in the office and bad morale. Production is eventually going to go down and people will leave the practice. They will be less focused. There will be a lot of careless-ness, because they are just too busy. One of the main priorities of the Practice Promoter is to make sure that the amount of Bonus Board activity is not placing too much strain on the team members.

Trait #5 – Personal Developer

❏ The Practice Promoter needs to get every member of the team to take ownership of their job and the entire practice and its results. Now, how do you do that? How do you instill this team ownership? Not the easiest, but certainly the simplest way to do it is to help them choose tasks that not only reward them, but also stretch them a bit and help them feel like they are a big part of practice growth.

Trait #6 - Motivator

❏ The Practice Promoter must get the entire team excited about the growth potential about your practice. This is where you must be a bit of a psy-chologist. Creating staff motivation is a huge tal-ent. There are all kinds of motivation. There is intrinsic motivation. There is extrinsic motivation. Extrinsic is what we are all used to in the Silicon Valley System; bonuses. Intrinsic is a little bit different and is where you have such a pride in your job and such a pride in your ability to do the job that you motivated yourself to do a good job from the inside. It is the quality a lot of Practice Promoters will have. It is the quality that will probably be rare in the other employees of the practice. It takes a very special person to have this. When a person has it, they generally rise to a station in life that has a leadership role. This person is going to have an internal drive. They're going to have a sense of a job well-done without anybody having to tell them. They will have pride and ownership in their job title and their job descriptions.

Trait #7 - Troubleshooter
❏ The Practice Promoter must spot challenges and roadblocks before they become too serious. It is the Practice Promoter's job to realize the trends that are going bad in the wrong direction and to help that doctor give them good ideas to find the roadblocks that are stifling practice growth. The team leader must then be open to creativity and new ideas. They must be able to talk to the doctor about those things and help form new solutions. The Practice Promoter cannot be afraid of change. Change is what makes the practice grow and helps to get off plateaus.

Trait #8 – Executive Assistance

❑ The Practice Promoter must take the managerial role of project completion off the doctor. What that does is it lessens the stress on the doctor. The team Practice Promoter must cease to be dependent on constant inspections by the doctor. They must be able to work on their own. When important non-clinical tasks are taken off the doctor's plate, the doctor can focus on the patients during the practice day and nothing else. This allows the doctor to have confidence and know that his choice of Practice Promoter is making his vision a reality. Eventually, the doctor gets to the point where the doctor no longer thinks about all those other things that used to bother them. The things that used to make dentistry more stressful than it should have been. The doctor can focus on the patient and do the thing that they were trained to do. Then the doctor can have the fun job of having the vision for the practice and helping the Practice Promoter stay on course with their vision. It is a win/win for everyone.

Practice Promoters are so tremendously important for a practice and especially a practice that is hoping to grow and achieve a vision.

Those are the eight rules for Practice Promoters and I hope everybody takes those to heart. To make it really con-crete in your mind, write them down and post them on the walls of your office. If you have a Practice Promoter, make sure those are burned into their brain. Having a quality Practice Promoter will make your practice and your life so much better.

CHAPTER TEN
HERE'S WHAT I LEARNED FROM THE DESTRUCTION OF MY OLD LIFE AS A DENTIST

On a stormy night in May, a lightning bolt came for me, and my life has never been the same.

The call came at 9:00 p.m. on a Tuesday.

The concern in my wife's voice triggered me to look up from my laptop. All the worst case scenarios raced through my mind.

Death in the family? Are the kids O.K.? What is wrong?

My wife put the phone down and said, "Your office is on fire."

I bolted off the bed and jerked on my tennis shoes. I was strangely calm; I suppose this stemmed from gratitude that the call hadn't brought much worse tidings. Still, my practice was my livelihood for me and for my family. Plus, the proud members of Griffin Dental who needed their paychecks to continue as scheduled weighed on my mind as I sped the two miles to my standalone 7,000 square foot dental practice.

A storm had blown through a few minutes earlier, and although the severe thunderstorms had subsided, a cold and steady rain came down as I approached the last curve in the road that led to my office.

It wasn't a long drive, but time for me had slowed to the point that I was able to run about a dozen scenarios through my mind. The worst case was a smoldering pile of rubble where my office once stood, and the best case was a huge misunderstanding, a few laughs with the responding emergency workers, and a trip back home to tell a funny story to my worried wife.

The two minutes it took to drive those two miles seemed like they lasted two hours. I topped the hill overlooking my practice and saw an eerie orange glow casting scary shadows on red fire trucks and scrambling volunteer firefighters in their yellow gear. I knew this was no misunderstanding. My office was on fire.

I parked next to a gargantuan Ripley Fire Department vehicle and leaped out into the madness. I found a firefighter and asked what I needed to do to help.

He urgently asked, "Where's the med gas?"

Med gas! Geez, that's right. If the fire were to hit the oxygen or the nitrous, we could have an explosion on our hands. That could level Griffin Dental, injure the first responders, and perhaps do a lot more damage to surrounding properties.

The firefighter and I raced to the back door close to my private office, and I started fumbling with my keys. I had to admit that I had left home in such a rush that I didn't have the key to that door.

Another firefighter pushed us aside and shouted in heroic fashion, "I don't need a key!"

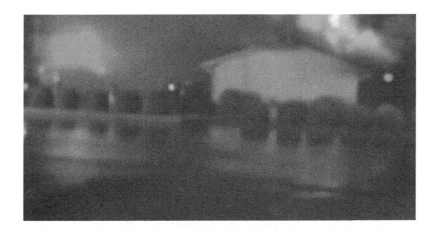

He kicked in the door the way you see guys like Bruce Willis or Vin Diesel do it in the movies. I didn't know they did that in real life until that night.

Thick, greenish-black smoke poured from the door as it broke inward, but the firefighter charged in anyway. Moments later he reemerged with a sick look on his face and went to his knees to vomit. The smoke was too much for him.

The fire captain shouted for his men to put on their oxygen masks. He asked me for explicit instructions on how to find the tanks of gas. I gave him a verbal map of the office, and the firefighters entered the burning building. In a minute or two they emerged from the flames, hauling out four large tanks of compressed gas. The tanks were scorched but intact.

Afterward, one of the firefighters would tell me that the closet where I kept the med gas had flames licking at the ceiling, and they had pulled out the tanks just in time. It was a truly heroic act, and it made me proud that regular people can put their lives at risk for the greater good of their community.

After that, there was really nothing left for me to do besides stand at a safe distance and watch my building burn. I stood at the corner of the parking lot, rain pouring down and soaking my clothes. My memory is a bit cloudy on the details. I think I entered a sort of trancelike state.

It was surreal watching the building that housed all my dental hopes and dreams slowly burn. I thought about how hard I had worked to succeed in my practice and to pay off the building's mortgage.

I didn't know what had caused the fire. Could it have been lightning? I wondered how well my insurance would cover my losses.

I wondered if the firefighters would somehow miraculously walk up to me and say, "Congratulations! We stopped the fire, and it shouldn't be that big a deal to fix up."

I wondered how long it would take me to pick up a hand piece and actually work on a patient again. If it took too long, would my patients leave me? Would my staff leave me?

Heck, if my insurance was really good, would I even want to work again? Maybe I should just ride off into the sunset and start a second career.

People started to parade past me as I stood there in the rain. Most wanted to say they were sorry. My dad and my wife came and tried to make me change my wet clothes. Most of my staff came by. I could see they were scared, but I was in no shape to console them.

I JUST STOOD IN THE RAIN, WATCHING MY PRACTICE BURN.

My mind was at war with itself in what could only be described as a true crisis of the soul.

I questioned everything I had done up to that one moment in my life, the moment that had interrupted everything.

I thought back to my days as an aspiring engineering student at Mississippi State, before the idea of dentistry had crossed my mind. I recalled my recruitment into the dental field and how my respected physician uncle had told me I was "wasting my life" going into a field like dentistry. Why had I still gone ahead? What had drawn me to the profession in the first place?

I thought about dental school and how hard it was, but I also remembered how the terrible difficulty of our coursework and clinicals had forged a lifelong bond with my classmates.

I recollected how I had made mistake after mistake in building my practice, but that I had eventually cracked the code and turned it into a Top 1% practice.

Would there be any clues left in the rubble to help me remember how we succeeded so well in the first place?

We had worked tirelessly to develop relationships with our patients. Would all that hard work be for nothing if we had to move?

Would we still be able to market successfully? Would anyone still want to be my patient if we were out of business for an extended period of time?

I didn't know the answer to any of these questions.

All I knew for sure right then was that 14 years of my life's work were smoking, smoldering, and falling down.

My only option at that moment was to stand in the rain and wait for the fire to stop.

At midnight, the fire died.

COULD I RISE FROM THE ASHES AND RECLAIM MY PRACTICE?

Weeks later I would learn that it was, indeed, a bolt of lightning that had struck my building and changed the course of my future in dentistry.

Even though I knew things would never be the same, I didn't make a decision on my future that fateful Tuesday night. I didn't have all the facts, and as I look back, the days immediately after the fire were a blur.

When it became obvious that my practice was beyond repair and had to be demolished, I was forced to make the big decision. Do I rebuild? Do I move? Do I start a new career and leave dentistry behind?

On Tuesday night, I didn't even know the right questions to ask.

On Thursday, I made the decision.

What happened on Wednesday? I discovered the right questions to ask.

Sometimes to find the right answers in life, you have to step away from the insanity that is the daily routine for most of us.

That fire may have turned out to be the biggest blessing in my life.

Why? Because it pushed the biggest reset button in my professional existence.

It allowed me to remove all the little built-up obstacles that had formed in my dental practice over 14 years like the tiny barnacles that attach to the bottom of an aging fishing boat.

I had the cleanest of slates, and I wanted to make sure I took full advantage of my opportunity, not only for myself but also for all my colleagues out there who are in a self-imposed jail cell of unhappy success.

Once all the noise and chatter of "the way things always have been" and "but if I do that ..." were removed, the only truly important questions came to me like a voice from above. They were:

❑ Am I happy in my life?
❑ Do my patients believe in me?
❑ Am I at peace with my future?

That's it. Three questions. Three yes or no questions at that, but they held the keys to all the things I hold dear and important.

On Wednesday, those three questions came to me like a light in the darkness.

The answers to those questions didn't come quite so quickly, and at first I didn't like the answers.

It wasn't until I lived through my dark night of the soul that I was able to face the reality of my situation and take charge of my future. I realized that I needed to take the first step toward a practice and a life that really mattered, for that was the only way I could answer yes to all three of those questions. I had to matter to myself, to my wife, to my family, to my friends, to my team, and to my patients.

While we struggled to rebuild the practice, my team and I were forced to work in a cramped 1,200 square foot former nurse practitioner's office that we converted into five ops. Without all of the luxury items to which we had been accustomed in our old building, things got tense in a hurry. We were literally bumping into each other most of the time. Worse than the internal struggles was the realization that many patients who I had assumed would be loyal, lifelong members of our practice found the seven extra miles they had to travel too much of a burden. Many were lost to other practices, and my hours at the chair dwindled. We couldn't produce at the same levels we achieved prior to the fire. My team's income dropped, meaning I froze their wages at the level they were in the months before the fire, temporarily eliminating bonuses, which I thought was exceedingly fair considering the way I was personally bleeding cash and fighting insurance companies. Over the next few months, I lost over half my employees, including some of my longest term staff members, representing more than 75 years of dental experience. It was heartbreaking to see people I cared about leave, especially knowing that even though they were too nice to say it, if I had been able to give them the bonuses they had come to expect, there's no doubt in my mind they would have stayed.

Not the loss of income or longtime patients but the loss of my dental teammates, my trusted allies in the fight to build a truly great dental practice, sunk me into the lowest point of my professional career.

We had been on a steady uphill climb for nearly 15 years, and several of my longest term employees had benefitted greatly from my belief in the death spiral bonuses I had learned from consultants in whom I had misplaced my trust. Those team members' departure from the practice hurt a lot. It was like losing a favorite aunt or cousin, only I spent a lot more time with my team members than with any of my non-immediate family members.

There's no doubt that all the heartache I suffered taught me some hard lessons that stuck with me and made me a better dentist, a better boss, and a stronger, smarter leader. When I was forced to start over, we hit on a winning system that I want so much to be able to share with all of you.

My goal for you is to have a dental team that handles everything for you so all you have to do is come in, be the doctor, and leave with peace of mind that everything is getting done. And that's not all. I want you to be surrounded by a happy, smiling staff that's more like a family than a group of coworkers.

I truly want you all to be able to make more, work less, and enjoy practice again. All of us deserve that and that's exactly what the Silicon Valley Bonus System can do for you.

STOP READING AND DO THIS NOW!

Yes, you read that right. What I am about to tell you is so important that you may need to put down this book and get on the phone to a computer backup service right now.

When the firefighters gave me the all clear to go into my burned dental office, what was the first thing I tried to save? My brand new CAD-CAM machine? Personal items such as family photos?

No.

I had to save my server. My server had all my practice data. My practice software, patient charts, schedules, X-rays, photos, you name it. I had to save that thing. When they gave me the signal, I rushed to the door closest to the server with my cousin and a firefighter. We found the server a little damp and smoky, but we were able to wrench it from the wall with the help of some cable cutters.

The next day my computer expert called with the bad news. When he opened the server, water ran out and the insides had melted from the heat. It was a total loss. How would I ever be able to recover all those years of patient information? That's it. My life as a dentist was over.

My computer expert broke into my depressing reverie. He had good news! He asked if I remembered him talking me into backing up my data off site about 10 months before. Honestly, I had forgotten all about it. My data had been backed up online every night for almost a year!

Three days after the fire, we had a temporary server loaded with all of our patient information and practice management software. If was as if an angel had reached into my burned-out building and pulled out a computer, intact. It became our lifeline as we set up practice in our temporary location.

I don't even want to count the loss to my hard-earned patient base if we hadn't had that data. If one of my colleagues asks me about getting online backup, I tell him or her to hang up the phone and call a service immediately. It is the best money I ever spent for my practice. Backing up our data literally saved us.

So, if you aren't backing up your practice data, stop reading. Go to the phone. Get back up. Do it now! Then come back to this book so you don't miss out on learning a brand new way to harness the most powerful team motivation tool ever created.

CHAPTER ELEVEN
IF YOUR DREAM PRACTICE WAS FOR SALE, WHAT WOULD YOU PAY TO OWN IT?

It is a very different practice than the one you are in today. Sure, the building is nice and modern. It's clean and neat, but that's not the real difference.

The staff is dressed neatly and seem busy, bustling around, but it's not chaotic. They even seen genuinely happy to be there.

No patients are ever ecstatic to come in for their dental procedures, but these patients seem peaceful and at ease. They kind of look like they are getting ready to visit with old friends.

There are no confrontations at the front desk over money or scheduling conflicts.

It's just different.

This practice already exists. The only problem is that right now it only exists in your mind and it is up to you to find a way to manifest your dream practice.

IMAGINE BUYING YOUR IDEAL PRACTICE.

What would it be worth to you? Can you imagine how awesome it would be to walk into your office each day and not feel like there are a million things that need doing that just aren't getting done? Stress kills. Can you imagine how much better your life would be without that stress? Can you imagine how long you could extend your practice life? What is that worth? Can you even put a price on it?

If you're thinking that you can't imagine the cost but that if it were possible to make that dream a reality, you would pay just about any cost, I have some great news.

Manifesting your dream practice is not impossible and it is not even expensive, it just requires doing things completely differently than you've ever done them before. The Silicon Valley System is a way of inspiring your team to action differently than any way that has been done in dentistry before. In the description laid out in this book, there are also clues to other ways you must act differently to make your dreams a reality.

If you want a different life, you must do things differently. Different than your peers at the dental society. Different than your friends at the class reunion. That's the hardest part of this book I think. I write this knowing that most readers will find it too hard to change for whatever reason. Whether it is an off-handed remark from another dentist about how there's no way it will work or a spouse who really doesn't understand the magic of taking action to change, most of you will take a small bit of inspiration from this book, but never make any real changes. Most don't really want to be different even if that's what it would take to succeed.

If you are one of the few brave souls who doesn't mind making powerful changes to be different, implementing the Silicon Valley Bonus System is the next obvious step towards making your dreams come true.

If you truly have the courage and drive to take that next step forward and make this system a reality in your practice, I can help because I have suffered through all the trial and error of perfecting the Silicon Valley Bonus System and have it down to a science.

How would you like to work with me directly so I can help you implement everything you just read about? That way, you won't have to go through all the headaches and hassles I went through.

IMPLEMENTATION

I have revealed the exact system we use in our practice every day, the system we have taught dentists all around the world to help build the practice of their dreams by tapping into the potential of a happy, motivated team. If you like what you've discovered here and want to take it to the next level, we have created a very special program where we not only help you form your own unique vision for your dream practice, but work with your team hand in hand as you install the Silicon Valley Bonus System in your own workplace. Plus, we have added a lot of really amazing bonuses to help you get started quickly. We call this program Team Leadership Class. If you're interested in taking the next step, head over here right now:

www.SiliconValleySystem.com
You'll be glad you did!

DON'T FORGET YOUR FREE
BONUS TRAINING WEBINAR

Register for your bonus training that goes with this book by going to **www.SiliconValleyBonus.com** On this training, you will learn:

- How to **identify a Death Spiral Bonus** before it makes everyone miserable and kills your team unity

- How to apply the Silicon Valley System to your Practice in a way that could <u>double your practice and make your team love you for it!</u>

- You can **stop spending THOUSANDS each year with big marketing companies and slick consultants** who try to convince you that your results are better than they actually are.

- This is THE MISSING PIECE of the training for Implants, CEREC, Ortho, or any other highly advanced skills you have acquired. I <u>don't even think you should do those trainings until you learn this protocol.</u>

- This is THE answer for the age-old problem of doctor›s not having enough time to manage their team. **The Silicon Valley Secret will turn you into a Lunch Hour CEO** (and it won›t even take nearly the whole hour.)

- Once Your team starts seeing how this makes the practice better, THEY WILL LOVE YOU FOR IT!

    Go to **www.SiliconValleyBonus.com** and sign up today

MEET DR. CHRIS GRIFFIN, DDS
DENTAL PRACTICE PRODUCTIVITY EXPERT ON A MISSION TO HELP DENTISTS WORK LESS, MAKE MORE, AND ENJOY PRACTICE ... AGAIN

Dr. Chris Griffin is a solo general dentist who focuses on work/life balance to be present for his family as much as possible. He graduated from the University of Tennessee in 1998 with a DDS degree and began solo practice in Mississippi in 1999.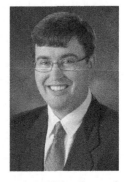

In 2007, Dr. Griffin was feeling the effects of the daily grind on his personal and professional life. That led him to cut his dental work week from five days per week to three days per week, starting in 2008. Much to his surprise, his practice grew by 20% that year even though he worked much less. This led him to found Capacity Academy to help other dentists learn the most efficient ways to perform dental procedures, focusing on general dentistry.

Since acquiring AGD PACE certification in 2009, Capacity Academy has hosted dental CE events with thousands of doctors attending Dr. Griffin's lectures all across the United States, and more than 100 doctors have traveled to his office in the tiny town of Ripley, Mississippi, for hands-on workshops.

HOW TO STREAMLINE YOUR CLINICAL SYSTEMS, OFFICE COMMUNICATIONS, SCHEDULING, AND PATIENT WORKFLOW TO MAXIMIZE EFFICIENCY

In his content-rich presentations, Dr. Griffin reveals how virtually any dentist can streamline systems and use inventive methods, such as color-coding and effective, common sense scheduling with a unique twist, so they can spend fewer hours treating patients each week and still maintain a vibrant, highly productive practice.

Chris wants dentists to discover an alternative to their daily, tiring grind and to enjoy peace of mind knowing they face a more certain future. He routinely helps dentists to improve their intra-office communication, speed up the patient treatment process, and be more productive while working fewer hours a week.

Now Dr. Griffin has another breakthrough to share with dentists. He has discovered a brand new way to harness the most powerful team motivation tool ever created ... a bonus system that works long term. Chris recently uncovered a secret that Silicon Valley technology giants use to motivate their teams, inspire innovation, and move projects seamlessly toward completion. He has converted this Silicon Valley secret into a bonus system that integrates with dental practices. In this book you will learn how to motivate and reward your team without creating a runaway monster bonus system that will eventually make everyone miserable and wreck your practice. When you implement the Silicon Valley Bonus System, you can turn your staff loose to build your practice and make your dreams come true.

Made in the USA
Monee, IL
04 October 2020